Practice Management Compendium

Part 1: Understanding the Contract

Practice Management Compendium

Part 1: Understanding the Contract
Part 2: Organising the Practice
Part 3: Finance and Reports
Part 4: Clinical Practices

Practice Management Compendium

Part 1: Understanding the Contract

by

John Fry

and

Kenneth Scott
General Practitioners

and

Pauline Jeffree
Practice Nurse,
Beckenham, Kent

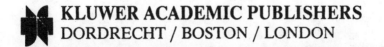

KLUWER ACADEMIC PUBLISHERS
DORDRECHT / BOSTON / LONDON

Distributors

for the United States and Canada : Kluwer Academic Publishers, P.O. Box 358, Accord Station, Hingham, MA 02018-0358, U.S.A.
for all other countries : Kluwer Academic Publishers Group, Distribution Center, P.O. Box 322, 3300 AH Dordrecht, The Netherlands.

ISBN 0-7923-8945-X

Published in the United Kingdom by Kluwer Academic Publishers, P.O. Box 55, Lancaster, U.K.

Kluwer Academic Publishers BV incorporates the publishing programmes of D. Reidel, Martinus Nijhoff, Dr W. Junk and MTP Press.

Origination by Roby Education Ltd, Liverpool.

Printed in Gt. Britain by Butler and Tanner Ltd., Frome and London.

Contents

Contents

Foreword

General Practice is undergoing the most major series of changes since the introduction of the National Health Service in 1948. They concern both concepts of care and practical details of the way care is delivered. In spite of the hostility generated by the changes most of the broad general concepts have been accepted. The principle of patients having more choice is widely supported, the inclusion of preventive medicine and anticipatory care in the responsibilities of practice has few opponents, the introduction of audit as a way of improving performance has been generally welcomed. Even the idea of putting GPs in better financial management of patients and drug budgets has had supporters in principle. The antipathy has generally related to the method of introduction of these changes. One important concern has been the time requirements of the New Contract and the feeling that these will erode the real nature of our work: the close personal relationship with patients.

If we improve the quality of our management this is less likely to happen. We shall be able to work within the New Contract and retain the quality of service we provide. If we improve the understanding of our staff of what we are trying to achieve we are more likely to reach the targets that we set whilst keeping people happy.

This book sets out to explain the New Contract. An understanding of this will be essential to those of us who have to work the system, and if we are better informed it will give us more chance of making the sensible amendments that will certainly be needed. I believe it will be a highly valuable source of information for Principals, Trainees and staff in practice and very strongly commend it.

Professor Sir Michael Drury
Head, Department of General Practice
University of Birmingham Medical School

Chapter 1

Background and Implications of the New Contract

HISTORICAL BACKGROUND

How and why has the new contract come about? To understand is to look back into the remote and the recent history of general practice.

There has always been a "healer of first contact", a primary health carer, to whom people went for help. Even Adam and Eve had each other! The first literature on general practice in Britain was written about 250 years ago when the healers were a motley collection of non-professionals, such as the local parish priest, the parish clerk, the Lady of the Manor, the "wise woman", the grocers and spicers and, of course, the itinerant quacks.

General practice was not recognised as a field worthy of a "college", although there had been colleges of surgeons and physicians since the 16th century. It was not until 1815 with the Apothecaries Act that the "surgeon apothecary" was recognised as a sort of physician of first contact who was allowed to dispense medicines. For the

...even Adam and Eve had each other...

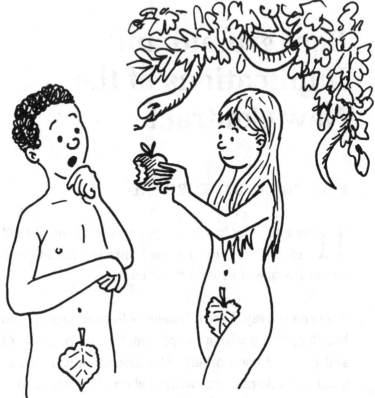

"'An apple a day keeps the doctor away'?
O.K. So what's the drawback?"

next 150 years the nameplates of GPs included the title of "physician, surgeon and accoucheur" and this aptly covered the field of work of a D.I.Y. doctor who was prepared to take on most conditions encountered, including most of the maternity work and much minor surgery. These doctors were paid fees or in kind, which was fine for those in wealthy districts, but not for those working with the poor.

This led to the beginnings of sorts of prepaid insurance schemes, such as sick clubs, organised by the doctor or some local agent, or larger groups, such as friendly societies, run by trade organisations and others.

In 1912 the National Health Insurance Act was piloted through Parliament by David Lloyd George, a minister in

...doctors were paid ...in kind...

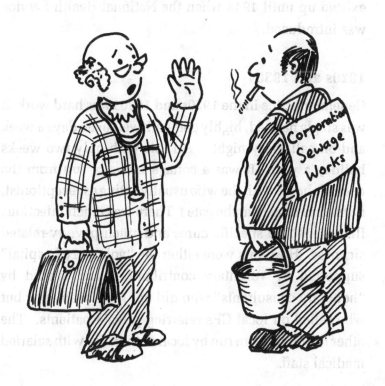

"No! No! I insist!
You can have this one on me"

the Liberal Government. The Act introduced compulsory insurance taxation, registration with a GP and regular payments by capitation.

The effects on general practice were t¹ at there were two groups of patients. One, "panel patients" who were on the panel for whom capitation fees were paid, i.e. working men and women, but their families were not covered. The others were "private patients" who paid fees for consultations, home visits and medicines. This system existed up until 1948 when the National Health Service was introduced.

1920s and 1930s

General practice in the 1920s and 1930s was hard work. It was single handed, highly competitive, seven days a week and on call every night . All this with only two weeks holiday a year. It was a cottage industry run from the doctor's home with the wife usually acting as receptionist, nurse and dragon at the gate ! There was much infectious illness with no specific cures and much poverty-related sickness. Hospitals were either the "voluntary hospital" supported by voluntary contributions and staffed by "honorary consultants" who did not receive any pay but who relied on local GPs referring private patients. The other hospitals were run by local authorities with salaried medical staff.

By this time it was becoming obvious that there was need for some form of national health service to cater for the less

...it was a cottage industry run from the doctor's home...

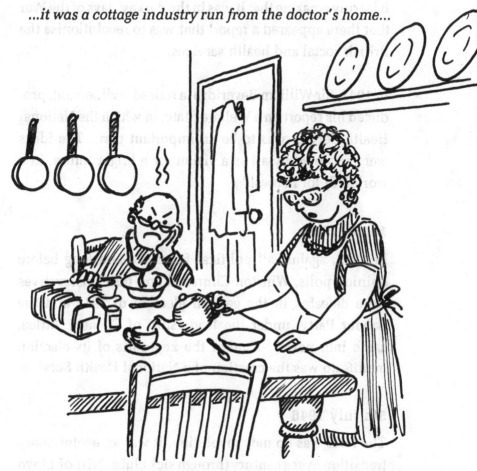

"Cottage industry it may be, but there'll be
no operations on *my* kitchen table!"

affluent and to promote better health. Both the government, usually Conservative, and the British Medical Association produced suggestions which were never followed up because of the impending World War II.

1939 - 1945: World War II

It is truly amazing that it was in the darkest days of the War that there appeared a report that was to revolutionise the British social and health services.

In 1942, Sir William Beveridge, a retired civil servant, produced his report on a Welfare State, in which the National Health Service was to be an important part. The ideas were accepted by all as a vision for a bright future, in a world "fit for heroes!"

1945 - 1948

In 1945, against all political forecasts, and long before opinion polls, Winston Churchill and his Conservatives were defeated in the general election of 1945 and the Labour Party, under the leadership of Clement Attlee, came into power. One of the key parts of its election manifesto was the creation of a National Health Service.

5th July 1948

The NHS was no new revolution, it was an evolutionary transition over a century through sick clubs, NHI of Lloyd George and traditional family practice developed over centuries.

Hospitals were nationalised but general practice, at first, was little changed. Patients registered with a GP, who was paid by capitation fees, and the local administration was the Executive Council, forerunner of the FPC. No longer was buying and selling of practices allowed.

On 5th July 1948 I (J.F.) experienced no changes with my patients, my premises, my staff (my wife) and my work. The major difference was relief that no longer did I have to charge fees and try to collect them and that I received a regular quarterly cheque.

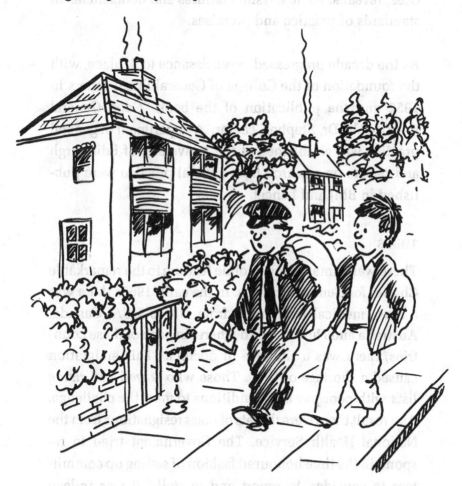

"The dogs are nothing. You should see a doctor if his cheque hasn't come"

1950s

The 1950s were times when general practice discovered itself. At the start of 1950 a report by an Australian, Dr. Joe Collings, in the Lancet, based on visits to 55 NHS practices, revealed some abysmal failures and deficiencies in standards of practice and premises.

As the decade progressed, a renaissance took place, with the foundation of the College of General Practitioners in 1952 and the publication of the book "Good General Practice" by Dr. Stephen Taylor. A department of general practice was established at the University of Edinburgh and papers on research from general practice were published in BMJ and Lancet.

1960s

These were times of low morale leading to the remarkable Charter for General Practice. In the early 1960s there was a mass medical emigration from UK to USA, Canada, Australia and New Zealand where, in each of these countries, there was a shortage of doctors. This emigration caused a shortage of GPs . Those who stayed had rising lists with poor pay and conditions to meet the challenge. As a result there were threats of mass resignations from the National Health Service. The Government tried to respond in the time honoured fashion of setting up committees to consider, to report and to stall. It was indeed fortunate for general practice that the four men in key positions were sensible men. Kenneth Robinson, the Labour Minister of Health, Sir George Godber, the Chief

...in the early 1960s there was a mass medical emigration...

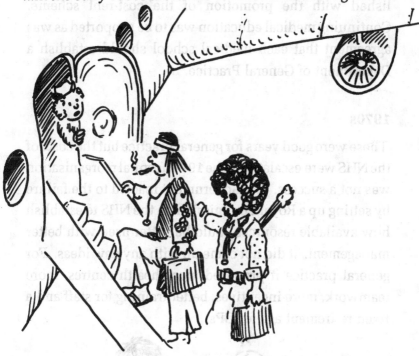

"Looks like another load of doctors."

Medical Officer and a friend of general practice, Ronald Gibson, a Winchester GP and Chairman of BMA Council and James Cameron, a Surrey GP and Chairman of GMSC. They got together over a few weekends and produced the Charter which transformed general practice.

Pay was to be increased through supplemental fees, group practice was to be encouraged through grants. 70% of staff salaries were to be reimbursed with a 100% reimbursement for rates and rent.

The General Practice Finance Corporation was established with the promotion of the cost-rent scheme. Continuing medical education was to be supported as was agreement that each medical school should establish a Department of General Practice.

1970s

These were good years for general practice but the costs of the NHS were escalating. The 1974 hospital reorganisation was not a success. The Government reacted to the failure by setting up a Royal Commission on the NHS to establish how available resources could be better used with better management. It did not come up with any new ideas. For general practice it proposed more health centres, more teamwork, more incentives, better training for staff and a fixed retirement age for GPs.

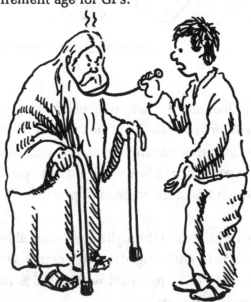

"Come off it, Methuselah! Early retirement at 780 isn't a bad offer."

1980s

The decade saw an attack on general practice with complaints from Community Health Councils and the House of Commons Select Committee on Social Services. Both supported the RCGP on the need to improve quality and service.

The Conservative Government, with a large parliamentary majority, applied its principles, of better value for money and privatisation, to general practice. Green and White Papers followed.

There was a lengthy period of secret back room negotiations between Government and BMA with the RCGP in the wings. These negotiations were inconclusive.

The confrontational negotiations were very different from the collaborative meetings that led to the Charter of 1965/6. On the Government side was a Secretary of State who was determined to have his way and who appeared to overwhelm his Chief Medical Officer, the Chairman of BMA Council together with the Chairman of GMSC. All three were unable to get their views accepted.

In the end the patience of the Secretary of State was exhausted and a new Contract was imposed on general practice.

There was a violent reaction from the profession but the Government won the day because of its huge majority in the House of Commons.

...confrontational negotiations...

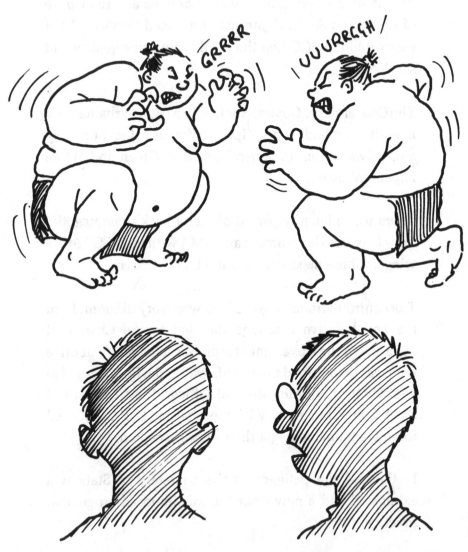

"I preferred it when we just used to sit down and talk."

Green and White Papers in the 1980s

1986

Primary Health Care: an agenda for discussion.
This Green Paper included most of the
principles that followed i.e. services more
responsive to consumer needs; raising
standards; promotion of health and prevention
of illness; giving patients more choices; FPCs
to have clear priorities; achieving better value
for money.

1987

Promoting Better Health. This was the White
Paper that enunciated government policies
along the lines of the Green Paper.

1989

Working for Patients. A fundamental White
Paper which covered future policies for the
whole NHS.

*General Practice in The National Health
Service: A New Contract.* Detailed
governmental proposals for changes to the
GP's terms of service and system of
remuneration.

IMPLICATIONS OF THE NEW CONTRACT FOR GENERAL PRACTICE

Whereas the 1965/6 Charter was better for general practice than patients, the New Contract was designed to do more for the public.

We shall detail its implications for general practice. Briefly it seeks to get much better value for money with more controls and directives and to provide better services for patients with more information and emphasis on disease prevention and health promotion.

1940 - 1990

The past 50 years have seen a flowering of British general practice relatively free to develop without too much interference from government.

Now with the imposed New Contract, life in general practice will be less independent and less free. It remains to be seen how many of its impositions will be viable, feasible and cost effective.

However, the New Contract is a fait accompli and we will need to consider how general practice can work it.

There are great difficulties for general practice. There have been no preceding tests nor trials of the proposed changes and no evaluation of the methods nor any attempts to test which are useful or useless. Neither has there been any real practical assistance or guidance on how they should be organised and implemented nor how problems may be anticipated and corrected. In this book we examine the New Contract in 3 parts :

- Services related to patients
- Services related to doctors and the practice team
- Services related to practice administration and organisation

For each item we discuss why it has been introduced and the thinking behind it, what is in it, and what effects it is likely to have on general practice. We make suggestions on how the practice can cope and where to seek assistance and advice.

What to do now

To meet the requirements of the New Contract it is essential for practices to have the fullest information about patients within each practice which, to date, has not proved necessary to run a well organised primary care service.

But !!

The parameters of general practice have now been extended by the Contract to such an extent that the new conditions can only be met by having the fullest details of the practice population.

Act now

Information is derived from data that is collected either manually or from computer. The maximum amount of data, with regard to basic patient information and practice activity, will have to be recorded to meet the demands made by the New Contract.

Manual collection

This can be achieved by the traditional establishment of a card indexed age - sex register which can be compiled from patients' existing practice records or from a computerised list of patients of the practice available from the FPC. Age-sex cards are available from the RCGP.

AGE - SEX CARD

Box 1	Indicate first or subsequent card
Box 2 - 8	Enter the number as on the doctor's prescription pad
Box 9 - 18	This is for the first 3 letters of the patient's surname plus the first initial of the first forename. The remaining component of the patient code is the full date of birth
Box 19	Male/Female
Box 20	Single, married, divorced, widowed or other
Box 21	Insert numerals 1 - 5 according to the Registrar General's classification of social groups.
Box 22 - 27	Insert date of entry to practice list
Box 28 - 33	Complete when patient leaves the practice
Box 34 - 35	Indicate reasons for removal from the list using FCP code
Box 36 - 61	Variable identification details relating to the patient e.g. 36 - 41 immunisation, 44 cervical smear

A.S.R.2a   **THE ROYAL COLLEGE OF GENERAL PRACTITIONERS**

Card	Dr. Code							Surname of Patient				Forename		Date of Birth			Sex	MS	SS
1	2	3	4	5	6	7	8	9	10	11		12		13–14	15–16	17–18	19	20	21

Addresses
1.

N.H.S. No. _____   F.P.C.

Date (Entry) _____ | 22–23 | 24–25 | 26–27 |

2.

Date (Removal) _____ | 28–29 | 30–31 | 32–33 |

3.

Reason _____ | 34 | 35 |

Occupation

Card to F.P.C.   /   /19

A	B	C	D	E	F	G	H	I	J	K	L	M	N	O	P	Q	R	S	T	U	V	W	X	Y	Z
36	37	38	39	40	41	42	43	44	45	46	47	48	49	50	51	52	53	54	55	56	57	58	59	60	61

A	B	C	D	E	F	G	H	I	J	K	L

SPECIAL INFORMATION

- 17 -

The age-sex register can be filed according to sex and in age bands so that cohorts of patients can be readily selected to provide the information that is required to meet the regulations of the New Contract:-

- new born for child surveillance
- children 0 - 5 years for immunisation
- well women 25 - 64 for cervical cytology
- patients over the age of 75 years for annual assessment.

Practices which have an up to date age-sex register will be able to readily identify the patients in these age bands.

Computer

Computerisation of patients' practice records is rapidly superseding the manual data collection system although it must be recognised that both systems need to be constantly updated to give reliable information.

Practices wishing to be computerised can obtain a download of the patient list from the FPC and this service should be available without charge.

There are several companies which produce software packages for general practice so that data can be refined to give all the information required to meet the needs of the New Contract.

Each target group can be "marked" in the computer system so that they can be audited at any time.

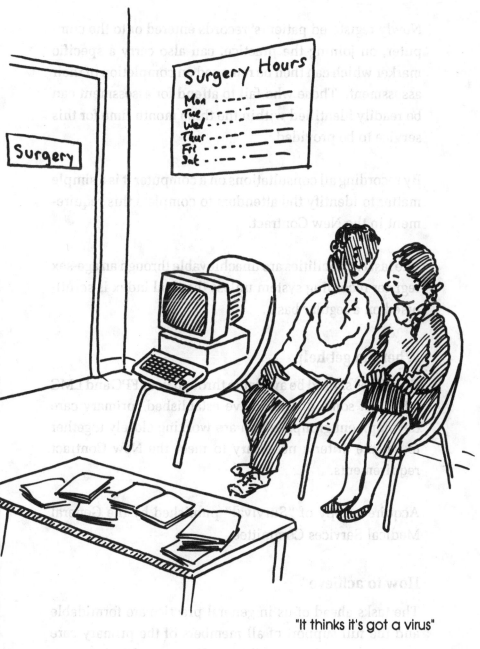

"It thinks it's got a virus"

Newly registered patients' records entered onto the computer, on joining the practice, can also carry a specific marker which can then be removed on completion of their assessment. Those who fail to attend for assessment can be readily identified within the three month time for this service to be provided.

By recording all consultations on a computer it is a simple matter to identify the attenders to complete this requirement in the New Contract.

The last two facilities are unachievable through an age-sex register recording system unless the total index is scrutinised on a regular basis.

Where to get help

Help lines should be available through your FPC and LMC which in some districts have established primary care development groups which are working closely together to set the criteria necessary to meet the New Contract requirements.

Acquire a copy of "Survival" published by the General Medical Services Committee.

How to achieve

The tasks ahead of us in general practice are formidable and the full support of all members of the primary care team is essential to meet the requirements of the contract, both to obtain the essential information and to devise systems for the information to be continually updated.

The practice manager should arrange meetings with the partners and the senior staff to identify needs and allocate tasks. There must be effective systems of communication within the practice to disseminate this information.

Who should do what ?

The new services we are expected to undertake will require considerable organisation and allocation of time. The co-ordination of these activities will rest with the Practice Manager, who forms a link between the professional and other members of staff in the practice.

The practice manager should arrange meetings with all members of the primary care team and practice support staff to identify needs for each programme to be undertaken by the practice. The manager must ensure that there are effective systems of communication within the practice so that each member of the team has a definite role to play in each of these new procedures expected to be undertaken in general practice.

The manager should also accept responsibility for organising appropriate training for all members of the practice. The major tasks which will need to be co-ordinated are listed overleaf.

Some tasks of the practice manager....

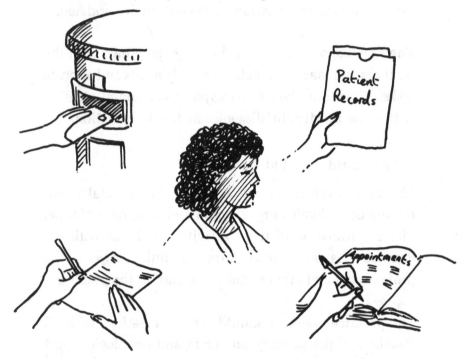

All members of the team need to meet and agree as to which procedures they wish to undertake in the practice, apart from those which are mandatory. They should agree who is to take the lead in each of these programmes. The GP must accept overall and full responsibility for the undertaking of mandatory tasks and accept referrals from other professional members of the team.

The practice nurse will play a major role in carrying out most of the programmes identified in the Contract. The nurse will need to follow agreed practice protocols and have certificates of competence should the tasks be part of an extended role from general nurse training.

Practice Managers Should Co-ordinate :

- accurate comparison of the list of patients held within the practice compared to that held by the FPC

- preparation of a practice leaflet giving full details as shown in Appendix 2

- devising of an accurate system to record practice activity and hospital referrals to be included in the practice annual reports to be published by June 1991 (Appendix 3)

- registration of new entrants - assessment examination offered

- recording of new births for child surveillance and immunisation programmes

- system for identifying patients who have not attended for a medical consultation in the past 3 years, so that these patients can be invited to attend the practice for screening

- recording of the assessment of 75 year old patients, and over, and to record whether assessments were undertaken in the patient's home or in the surgery

- identification of those health promotion clinics which the practice wishes to undertake

- planning of minor surgery sessions for those practices wishing to gain approval to undertake surgical procedures

- identification of a programme for call and recall of women patients eligible for cervical cytology. This service should be incorporated into a "well woman clinic"

The receptionists are the first point of contact with the patient within the practice. They play an important role in introducing patients to the new programmes of care. It would be hoped that their introduction to the new services would encourage patients to attend e.g. new entrants' screening.

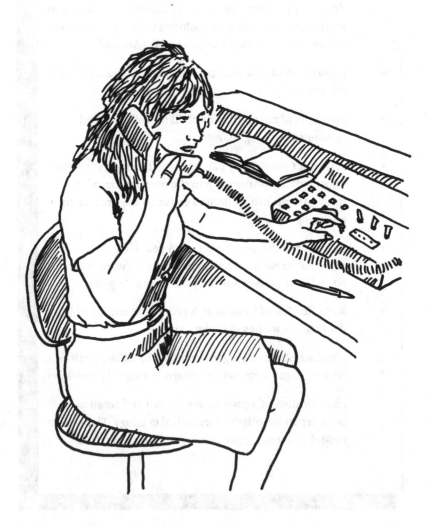

Clerical staff will be responsible for sending appropriate letters giving firm appointments for patients to attend the practice programmes for which they have enrolled. It must be recognised, at this early stage of the implementation of the New Contract, that the need to keep accurate data about all practice activities is essential for short and long term planning.

Chapter 2

Services Related to Patients

DOCTOR'S AVAILABILITY

The Contract specifies the amount of time that a general practitioner has available for patient consultations and of how patients will be informed of the time.

Why Introduced ?

It appears that behind the reasoning was the belief that some doctors have not, in the past, been available to their patients for sufficient hours because of other professional commitments or non-professional activities outside of the practice. It was felt that perhaps general practice had become a part time occupation and that the NHS was not getting sufficient value for money.

It was believed that the traditional independent entrepreneurial status of a general practitioner was too free and without sufficient specified conditions for the paymasters.

It was also believed that the services of general practitioners, their availability and consulting hours were arranged more to suit the doctors than their patients.

Associated with such thinking have come demands for information to be given regarding the availability to patients of doctors and other members of the practice team. For example, details of appointment times and out of hours cover should be made public through leaflets. Implied also, is that patients or their representatives should be able to be involved in such matters.

What is in the New Contract ?

It is expected that doctors should be available -

- on 5 days in a week, unless approval by the Family Practitioner Committee for 4 days by virtue of the doctor undertaking health related services on the unavailable day

- for not less than 26 hours in any week for consultations in the practice (this does not include travel time or other tasks) unless special arrangements for less have been made with the FPC

- for 42 weeks in any 12 month period

What effects ?

The effects of such directives can be seen in likely numbers of consultations and time spent on them by a typical NHS general practitioner.

- the average list size per NHS GP now is 2000 patients

- the mean number of consultations per person registered is 4 per year

- therefore there will be 8000 consultations during the year - 7200 or more in the surgery and 800 or less in home visits

- this means approximately 160 per week, for a year, or 32 per day

- allowing 10 minutes per consultation/home visit, the amount of time spent by the GP will be 27 hours per week, or 5.5 hours per day

Of course, this analysis only applies to standard consultations.

In addition, as will be seen from other expectations of the GP in the New Contract, the doctor will be expected to be involved in practice administration and continuing education; in child surveillance; maternity care; health promotion; examination of all new registrants; examination of all 3-year non-attenders and all those patients over 75 year of age to be visited each year.

The amount of time that these additional tasks can take will add considerably to the basic weekly 27 hours of consulting time, perhaps as much as 10 - 15 hours.

It must also be realised that many GPs have more than 2000 patients and a GP with 3000 patients can expect to spend 40 hours a week, or 8 hours a day, merely in consultations.

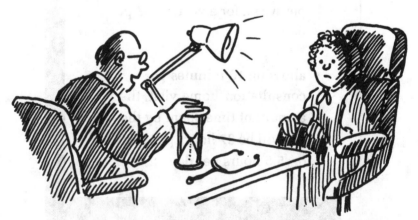

"You have 2 minutes, Mrs Clegg, on your complaint, starting.....NOW!"

CHANGING DOCTORS

Since November 1989 it has been made easier for patients to change their GP.

Why Introduced ?

The reasons were that it was assumed that there were many dissatisfied NHS patients who have found previous regulations frustratingly bureaucratic in changing from one GP to another.

No good evidence was provided on the extent of such dissatisfaction. Probably it amounts to less than 1% of patients in any practice at any time.

The essence of good general practice is to promote long term personal doctor-patient care rather than to encourage "shopping around" among GPs.

What is in the New Contract ?

It is now possible for NHS patients to change their GP -

- without prior consent from their present GP
- without seeking authority from local FPC
- with immediate effect.

Women receiving maternity medical services and children registered for health surveillance can also change GP without prior consent.

It must be noted that if a GP is not prepared to accept a patient onto the practice list, the doctor is still, nevertheless, responsible for providing immediate necessary treatment for which a fee can be claimed.

It is not stated whether a GP can remove a patient from the list immediately and without prior notice.

What Effects ?

The extent of the effects of this change will be minimal because, as previously noted, probably less than 20 patients a year, per GP, will change doctor in this way.

The wider issues raised will be of more concern-

- why do patients wish to change ?

- which patients and which doctors ?

- will such patients be able to obtain easy acceptance by other GPs ?

NEW REGISTRANTS

I t is directed that all newly registered patients (over 5 years of age) should be offered a consultation and examination.

Why Introduced ?

It has to be accepted that it is good practice to meet and get to know patients. Until now it had been left to the patients to come and see their doctor as and when necessary.

The New Contract imposes on the GP an instruction that all such newly registered patients should be seen and examined. The reasoning is that, in addition to a doctor-patient meeting, it will offer opportunities for health promotion, for screening and early diagnosis, checking on treatment being taken and for information to be given about the practice.

What is in the New Contract ?

The New Contract instructs GPs to offer a consultation to all new patients joining their lists who are over 5 years of age and provided that they have not been on a list of a partner within 12 months.

The GP is required to write to the newly registered patient offering a consultation within 28 days of acceptance to the list. If the patient is unable to attend the practice premises, then a home visit should be offered.

A sample letter of invitation is contained in Appendix 4

A record in the patient's notes must be made of the offer and as to whether it has or has not been accepted.

The consultation and health check can be delegated to a suitably trained member of the practice team.

The protocol to be followed should include -

- medical history
- check on medication
- lifestyle screening
- measurements of height, weight, blood pressure and urinalysis for sugar and albumen

The fee can be claimed providing that the consultation has taken place within 3 months of registration, or by special arrangement with the FPC for up to 12 months.

What Effects ?

It is likely that about 10% of the practice patients may move in or out each year. This means that there will be approximately 200 new registrants over the age of 5 years.

If all are to be seen and examined it means 4 - 5 each week at about 20 - 30 minutes for each consultation this will involve at least 2 hours work each week. Not only will this take up time, but it is likely that more work will be generated.

It is quite uncertain how many newly registered patients will respond to the invitations. This poses the question as to what sort of lengths should the practice go to chase up non-attenders.

In any event there will always be difficulty in arranging mutually convenient times.

...what sort of lengths should the practice go to chase up non-attenders...

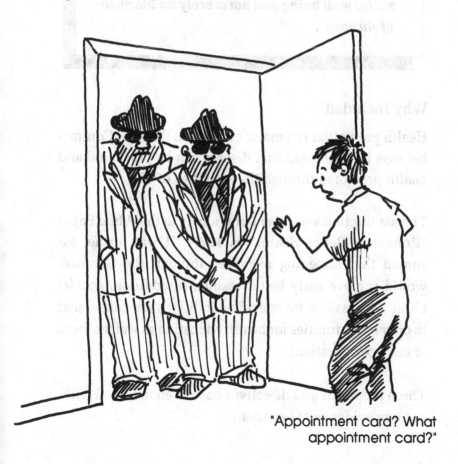

"Appointment card? What appointment card?"

HEALTH PROMOTION

The World Health Organisation's definition of health is "a state of complete physical, mental and social well being and not merely an absence of disease".

It is towards this utopian goal that promotion of better health is being pushed into the orbit of general practice.

> *"..a state of complete physical, mental and social well being and not merely an absence of disease".*

Why Included ?

Health promotion is a major concept in the New Contract because it is assumed that disease can be prevented and health promoted through the activities of GPs.

The assumption was raised previously in the White Paper "Promoting Better Health" in 1987. It was further assumed that screening exercises through the GP team would achieve early better results; in addition, special clinics or sessions for specific conditions are considered to offer opportunities for health education as well as those at each consultation.

These proposals and directives have been included without any evidence of benefits.

What is in the New Contract ?

A new sessional fee will be available for practice health promotion clinics. There has to be approval from the local FPC for type of clinic, its frequency, numbers attending and who should conduct it.

The types of subjects considered suitable are :-

- well person clinics - men and women
- heart disease prevention clinic
- diabetes clinic
- lifestyle clinic

including : -
- anti-smoking
- alcohol control
- stress management
- exercise counselling

The practice will be expected to advertise its clinics through practice leaflets, and FPC directories available in public places, and to invite its patients through personal invitations.

For approval, each session should last at least one hour, include at least 10 patients for a group, but that health promotion can be provided individually as well as in a group - FPC approval should be obtained.

For success, there should be practice guidelines to be agreed and followed -

- practice staff should be motivated to agree that clinics are worthwhile

- agreement should be obtained on the subject and programme, procedures, methods and guidelines

- practice staff and patients should understand their respective roles and targets to be achieved

- resources required must be defined, space allocated and costs estimated and funded

- groups of patients should be targeted, their names and addresses checked, invited and followed up

What Effects ?

This could become a major component of general practice work. If all the listed clinics were to be undertaken in a group practice of 4 GPs, it is possible that two clinics may be required each week at 1 - 2 hours each. Much time would also be taken up in administration, organisation and, of course, costings.

CHILD SURVEILLANCE

The field of observing development of children has made great advances over the past 25 years and has added much to our knowledge of what is normal and of what is abnormal.

Why Included ?

The New Contract group believe that child surveillance is so important that GPs should be encouraged and motivated to carry out this exercise on all children in their practices.

Good childcare has to start before birth and the GP antenatal clinic is the place where preparation for child care should start through health education from, and contact with, the health visitor who is going to relate to the mother after the birth. There is no mention of antenatal care in the New Contract.

The precept is that one object of surveillance is early diagnosis of correctable physical conditions such as congenital dislocation of the hips, undescended testes, cardiac abnormalities, eye disorders, deafness, scoliosis and slow mental development.

There are other possible advantages in promoting better GP/mother, health visitor/mother relationships.

What is in the New Contract ?

GPs are "encouraged" to undertake Child Surveillance in their practices and part of that encouragement is that it attracts service fees for children 0 - 5 years.

To obtain the fee, form FP/CHS has to be submitted for each child for whom the service is to be provided.

Approval of FPC has to be obtained for the GP to be allowed to carry out reimbursable Child Surveillance, and the doctor will be expected to have had experience and received training in this field.

What Effects ?

To carry out Child Surveillance, facilities have to be available, time has to be set aside and there should be a time set aside for collaboration with the health visitor .

For each GP with 2000 patients there will be 25 births in a year. The Child Surveillance programme will involve up to 5 examinations for each child in the first year of life. In addition, there will be 3 attendances for immunisations in the first year. This means in the first year -

- 5 attendances for Child Surveillance
- 3 attendances for immunisation
- ? attendances (some up to 5) for medical problems

This means 125 attendances (25 x 5) per GP for Child Surveillance in the first year at 15 - 30 minutes each, or 1 - 2 hours each week.

The income generated for Child Surveillance per GP, with a list of 2000 patients, will be about £480.00 per year, or about £4.00 per examination.

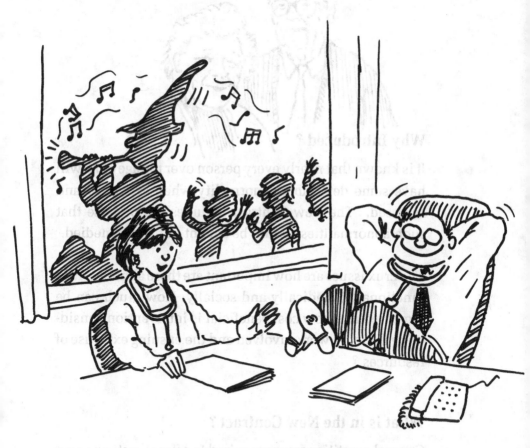

"So what's this bright idea of yours to get the kids along to clinic?"

HEALTH CHECKS FOR PATIENTS OVER 75 YEARS OF AGE

Most people over 75 years of age are active and able to enjoy a good quality of life. Some believe that they should also be free of all detectable abnormalities.

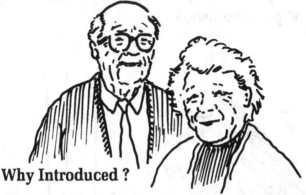

Why Introduced ?

It is known that nearly every person over the age of 75 will have some detectable abnormality when examined and assessed. The New Contract includes the premise that such abnormalities should be sought out and remedied.

The crux issues are how important are these abnormalities functionally, medically and socially. How much can be remedied and how cost beneficial is intervention considering the extra work involved and the ensuing extra use of resources ?

What is in the New Contract ?

General practitioners are required to offer all patients over the age of 75 years an annual consultation and/or a home visit to assess whether any personal medical services or social services are required.

The offer should be made before 1/04/91 for the first round. It should be made in writing and a note made in the patient's records, together with the response, findings and actions. The assessment can be delegated to the practice nurse or health visitor.

A sample letter of invitation is contained in Appendix 5

ASSESSMENT FOR PATIENTS OVER 75

- general health
- copability
- sensory functions, i.e. sight and hearing
- mobility
- mental condition
- physical state including -

  continence

  pressure

  weight

  height

  urinalysis

  social environment

  current medical problems

  medication (and compliance)

  smoking

  alcohol intake

What Effects ?

There are many problems involved in carrying out this part of the New Contract -

POTENTIAL PROBLEMS e.g. how to:

- target the group and how to make contact

- arrange the consultation and/or home visit

- record the information

- arrange follow up for any care that may be required i.e. referral to medical or social services

- ensure acceptance and compliance

- check outcome/benefit

- cope with the extra work

About 6.5% of a practice population are over 75, or 130 in a practice of 2000. Approximately 80% of these will consult or be visited at home in any one year.

If all the 130 are to be seen in a year, then it requires about 3 consultations/home visits per week at 30 - 60 minutes each if the full assessment is to be carried out, or up to 2 hours a week.

It has to be questioned whether such expenditure of time and resources, including those that will have to follow many of the assessments, are worth the efforts.

HEALTH CHECKS FOR PATIENTS NOT SEEN WITHIN 3 YEARS

Most patients who do not consult can be assumed to be "healthy" or coping with their problems. There is no good evidence to the contrary.

Why Introduced ?

The New Contract assumes that the above hypothesis is not the case and that patients who have not consulted for 3 years may have hidden and unsuspected disorders that require prompt diagnosis and prompt treatment.

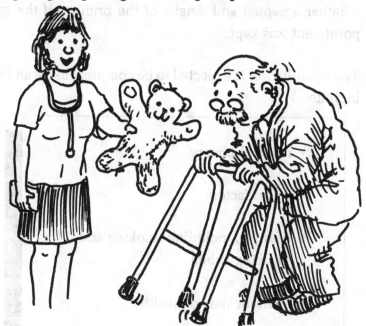

"Long time, no see, Mr Scoggins.
You left this on your last visit."

What is in the New Contract ?

For no extra fees, under the terms of service in their New Contract, the GP is obliged to offer a consultation to every patient aged 16 - 74 years who has -

- had no consultation for 3 years with any doctor
- had no "health check consultation" in the previous 12 months

Invitations for a consultation are expected to be sent out in writing to all those in the category before 1/04/91, and records kept of the date when the invitation was sent out, whether accepted and details of the findings if the appointment was kept.

The consultation is expected to be comprehensive and to include:-

- medical history

- social factors

- lifestyle, including smoking and drinking habits

- "current state of health"

- measurements of height, weight, blood pressure and urinalysis

The findings are to be recorded in notes, discussed with the patient and appropriate actions taken if necessary.

The GP is expected to inform FPC if a patient is not living at the registered address.

The result of patients not notifying a GP of a change of address is bound to cause great problems with -

- picking out 3-year non-attenders
- sending out invitations
- non-acceptance of invitations
- arranging mutually appropriate and convenient times for consultation
- cost and resources of the exercise (all at no extra fees !)

About 15 - 20% of adults (aged 16 - 74) will not consult over 3 years. This means 300 - 400 per GP with 2000 patients.

It means that in a year for the exercise to meet the terms of the Contract :-

- 6 - 8 will have to be seen each week each consultation will take over half an hour
- 3 - 4 hours will be required each week plus administration (at no fee!)

MINOR SURGERY

Traditionally, and pre-NHS, GPs nameplates read "physician, surgeon and accoucheur". Minor, and not so minor, surgery was very much part of general practice. Since the NHS, it has become a rarity for a few enthusiasts.

Why Included ?

Possible reasons must include :-

- saving of money, because it is believed that minor surgery in general practice is cheaper than in hospital

- promoting skills of GPs and making work more interesting

- promoting GP/hospital relationships

- promoting better GP/patient relationships

However, there are considerable problems that have to be faced, particularly those of competence, quality and safety, as well as those of organisation, expenditure and costs.

What is in the New Contract ?

Minor surgery by GPs is encouraged. Before a GP can be remunerated for the work, approval has to be gained from the FPC with regards to the doctor's experience and suitability of premises and facilities.

A list of procedures eligible for a fee are contained in Appendix 6.

The GP will receive a fee of £120.00 for carrying out 15 listed surgical procedures each quarter. The fee will be paid on a sessional basis, a session consisting of at least 5 procedures, not necessarily at one single session as they can be spread out during the quarter.

A GP is eligible for only 3 sessions a quarter, or 1 per month, but if the doctor is in a group practice claims can be made for more procedures on behalf of partners, i.e. for 3 sessions per partner per quarter.

What Effects ?

Thus each GP will be paid £120.00 for 15 surgical procedures in a quarter, or 60 a year, at the rate of £8.00 per operation, or £480.00 a year.

...there are considerable problems....particularly those of competence, quality and safety...

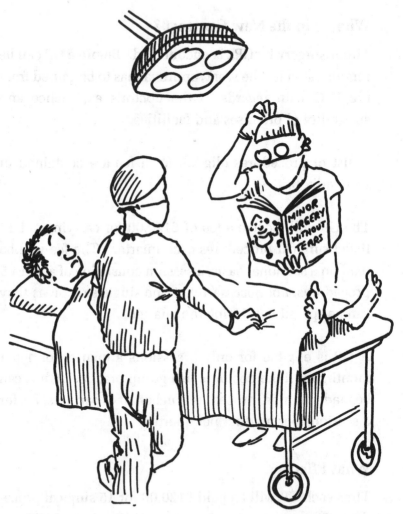

"I told you that you'd turned over 2 pages.
You've just performed the world's first
ingrowing vasectomy"

It is likely that taking in all costs to include nurse's time, equipment, premises etc., the cost to the practice per surgical procedure is £20.00

Allowing at least 30 minutes per procedure each session will take about 3 hours.

Chapter 3

Services Related to Doctors

DEPRIVATION ALLOWANCE

On the assumption that a GP in a "deprived area" has more work, more difficulties and more stress, it has been decided to compensate such doctors with extra supplementary capitation for each patient on their list.

What is it ?

Scales of deprivation are based on the Jarman Index (Brian Jarman is Professor of General Practice at St Mary's Hospital Medical School, London). Jarman devised a system of scoring social factors to measure "deprivation".

Ten social factors are used to produce scores. The present index is based on the 1981 Census, the next one being in 1991. It is likely that there have been considerable changes in some areas.

Three levels of deprivation payments are to be made - maximum, medium and minimum - to be, as noted, a supplement to the capitation fee for each patient on the

THE SOCIAL FACTORS MEASURED ARE :

- pensioners living alone

- children under 5 years of age

- single parent families

- unskilled bread-winners

- unemployed

- overcrowded households

- mobile populations denoted by high removal rates

- households with ethnic minority groups

- over 65s

- lack of amenities

practice list and living in the designated area. Therefore, GPs should ensure that addresses are accurate in order to qualify for payment.

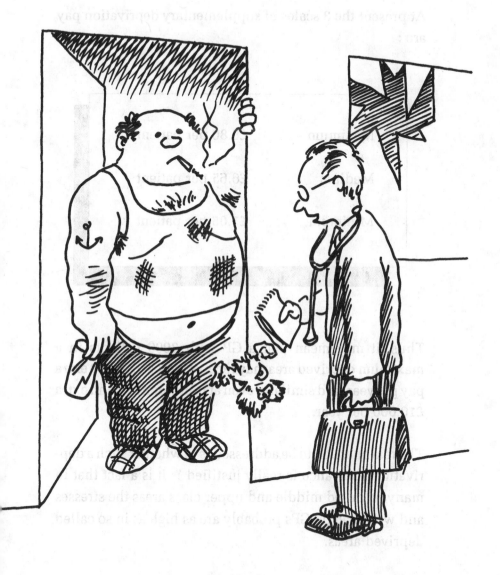

"well I suppose my address list could
be wrong. Are you *sure* you're not the
Duke of Westminster?"

What Effects ?

At present the 3 scales of supplementary deprivation pay
are :

Maximum	£8.80 per patient
Medium	£6.65 per patient
Minimum	£5.05 per patient

Thus, it may mean that a GP with 2000 patients in a
maximum deprived area may receive almost £18,000 extra
pay per year, and similarly even at minimum scale an extra
£10,000 per year.

The real question to be addressed is to whether such a deprivation allowance is really justified ? It is a fact that in
many so called middle and upper class areas the stresses
and workload on GPs probably are as high as in so called
deprived areas.

NIGHT VISITS

Night visiting by GPs has always been an integral part of general practice. It has disappeared in many other countries where it is carried out by a separate recognised group of doctors or where it does not occur at all, the patients making their way to hospital accident-emergency departments.

Why Included ?

The NHS has always rewarded night visiting as an unsocial task undertaken by GPs. This is retained in the New Contract, but a distinction is made between GPs carrying them out and a commercial deputising service doing the job.

What is in the New Contract ?

Two major changes have been introduced -

- the time span for a "night visit" has been increased by 2 hours, from 11 p.m. - 7 a.m. to a new time span of 10 p.m. to 8 a.m.

- differential payments for GPs carrying out their own night visits, or in a group or rota of up to 10 local GPs, which attract much higher rates of over £45.00 per night visit, and those carried out by commercial organisations at a much lower rate of around £15.00 per night visit.

What Effects ?

It is likely that with the extra 2 hours, a GP with 2000 patients can expect 30 - 40 night visits per year, which averages out at less than 1 per week during a year. However, if in a rota more night visits will be carried out on the nights-on-call.

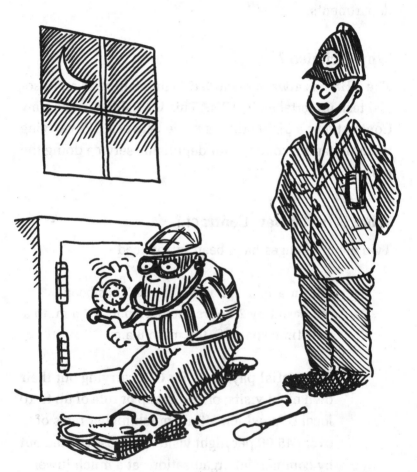

"How's its chest, then, Doctor?"

POSTGRADUATE EDUCATION

A more complex system of financial encouragement is introduced for GPs to undertake continuing learning in structured ways.

Why Included ?

Postgraduate education is considered essential for GPs. It should be noted that there are no such arrangements for consultants - is it that they are considered not to need such education or that they do not require such encouragement?

The Postgraduate Education Allowance is there to induce GPs to undertake continuing learning, to include subjects which are considered appropriate by the Department of Health, and for set amounts of time in specified ways.

What is in the New Contract ?

"Section 63" has been abolished and the new Postgraduate Education Allowance (PGA) includes monies to be spent on fees for courses. Market force principles have been introduced. GPs are expected to buy courses that they want, providing that they are approved and fit the proposed mix of subjects. The "PGA" will also be available for "expenses".

Presumably those educators who organise courses will be competing to sell their wares in a free market.

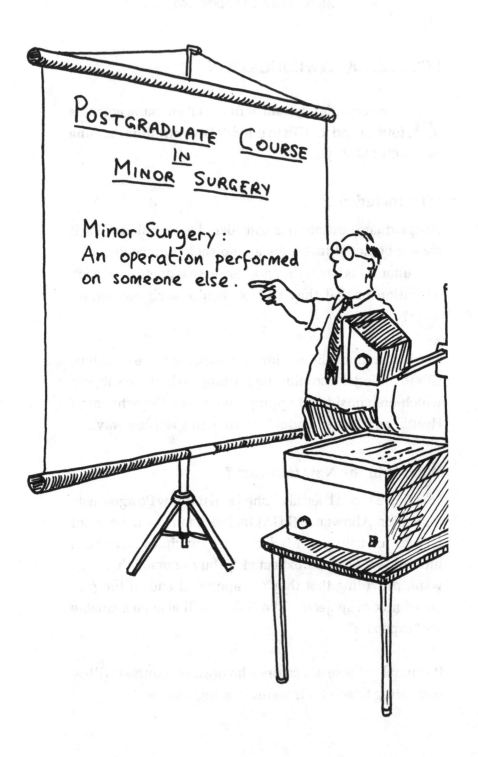

GPs are expected to -

- spend 25 days over a five year period in postgraduate education

- include specified amounts on courses in health promotion and disease prevention; in disease management; and in service management

The courses must be approved by the Regional Postgraduate Adviser, both in content and method. It is allowable for groups of GPs to arrange their own courses if the programmes are balanced and involve 5 GPs.

The busy New Contract GP will be expected to spend one working week a year in approved continuing education, or one whole day every 2 months, or a quarter of a session every week.

TARGET PAYMENTS

Rather than relying on simple fees for work done towards prevention, the New Contract proposes payment only when agreed targets are attained.

Why Included?

Target payments are intended to be incentives to achieve very high levels of immunisation for children and similarly very high targets for cervical cytology.

The objective is for GPs to carry out National Health policies.

The groups targeted in the present scheme are

> - children up to the age of 2 years and pre-school children for immmunisation
>
> - women 25 - 64 years (21 - 60 in Scotland) for cervical cytology

What is in the New Contract?

Differential rates of payments are set for targets to be achieved. Maximal rates will be paid for -

- complete immunisation for at least 90% of all children in their first 2 years, and for pre school children. Lower rates are paid for immunisation of 70% - 80%

- for at least 80% of women in any specified age group (excluding those who have had a hysterectomy) who have had a cervical smear and lower rates for 50% - 79%

What Effect?

There will be considerable problems in achieving the maximal rates, not only in providing the facilities for carrying out immunisation and cervical cytology, but also ensuring that those in the specified age groups take up the offers.

Good age-sex registers, recording, follow up, recall and information systems will have to be developed and maintained. The work load per GP with 2000 patients will involve -

- for immunisation 125 attendances by the 25 children in their first year, and the 25 in their second year of life: this means 3 - 4 per week or 1 hour per week

- for cervical cytology it will be necessary to carry out some 200 cervical smears every year per GP with 2000 patients, or 4 - 5 per week, or some 2 hours per week.

CHILD HEALTH SURVEILLANCE *(SEE ALSO PAGES 39-41)*

I t is generally accepted that, in many general practices, the attention to child surveillance will be carried out in close liaison with the health visitor.

Why Included ?

Modern belief is that child health surveillance is necessary to -

> • allow for support and general education of the parents
>
> • teaching the principle of good health to the whole family
>
> • detection of abnormalities and arranging for correction and management
>
> • recording normal progression of child development
>
> • promotion of immunisation
>
> • to provide financial incentives for GPs to carry out this work

What is in the New Contract ?

GPs must be approved to carry out child health surveillance and will be eligible only if they have undertaken the
appropriate training or had experience in the discipline
over the past 5 years.

They will have to follow local directives set by specialists,
as well as to record and report findings. There will probably be at least 7 - 8 surveillance examinations per child in
the first 5 years.

What Effects?

For a GP with 2000 patients there will be 125 children aged
0 - 5 years. With each child requiring 7/8 surveillance
examinations during this time means that there will be
200 examinations a year, or 4 per week at 2 hours a week.
These can be shared with health visitors.

Chapter 4

Developments in Practice Administration

COMPUTERISATION

The requirements of practices to fulfil their commitments under the new terms of service and the General Practitioner Contract are such that it will be essential to collect activity data about all aspects of their work.

This data is only of value when it is converted into information. This can best be achieved through the use of a computer.

Data will need to be refined to give the information that will be needed, e.g. to complete Practice Annual Reports.

There are several systems on the market and companies are producing both hardware and software to keep abreast of the change and, at the same time, are updating their equipment and data collecting systems.

It is anticipated that software will shortly be produced to assist practices in handling their indicative drug budgets.

Computerisation is a major commitment and is only as good as the information that is fed into the system. The reliability of the reports depends on the accuracy of the data recorded.

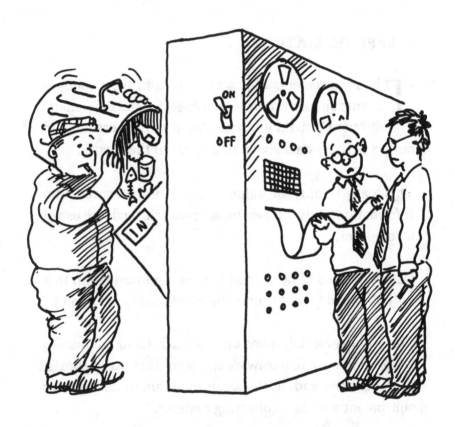

"I can't understand why all we seem to get out of it is garbage."

PRACTICE LEAFLETS AND ANNUAL REPORT

I t is mandatory for practices to produce practice leaflets and an annual reports

Practice Leaflets

Practice leaflets should give :

- full details of the doctors within the practice
- the roles of the staff with whom they work
- details of the facilities within the practice
- the surgeries and clinics which are provided by the practice

For full details of the requirements of practice leaflets see Appendix 2.

The object of practice leaflets is to keep the patients informed of services provided by their doctors, including the doctors' availability, details of qualifications and the service provision.

Annual Reports

General practitioners are expected to issue an annual report giving a comprehensive view of the previous year's activity and proposed changes for the following year.

The first report will cover the period from 1/04/90 to 31/03/91 and must be submitted to the FPC by 30/06/91.

The Annual Report will contain the following -

1. Staffing - speciality hours of work qualifications training experience.

2. Premises - any changes that have taken place in the premises and proposed changes for the ensuing 12 months.

3. Referral patterns - including - total number of patients directly admitted the number of patients referred to a hospital out patient department self-referral when this is known to the GP. For details of specialities to which patients have been referred see Appendix 3

4. Commitments - the doctors other commitments as a medical practitioner referring to the type of post and the description of the work undertaken, including the amount of time spent on these projects.

5. Drug information - whether or not the practice has its own formulary and the details whereby repeat prescriptions are issued to patients.

WHAT DOES IT ALL MEAN FOR GENERAL PRACTICE ?

The changes envisaged for general practice by the introduction of the New Contract and the variation of the terms of service are formidable and have major implications for every practice in U.K. The foresight behind these changes has considerable merit because it will raise firstly the standards of general practice from its historic, essentially unstructured, prescribing/diagnostic treatment service to a more meaningful primary care provision with emphasis on prevention.

Although the Government's approach has been somewhat dynamic in expecting dramatic changes to happen nationally in an incredibly short time, realistically these changes will be more gradual.

The restructuring of the Family Practitioner Committee into a new authority, with its own general manager, and subsequent reorganisation has significant bearing on the implementation of the New Contract. This Contract can be interpreted by each FPC which, hopefully, is being undertaken in consultation with its Local Medical Committee.

In the future FPCs will be obtaining their medical advice from a doctor who is unrelated to the district and hopefully that doctor will become acquainted with the needs of both doctors and patients in the district.

The detailed organisation of general practice and service planning that will need to be undertaken will have significant implications not only for the single-handed practitioner, but also for the smaller group practices.

The level of professional expertise that will be required to provide the data that is mandatory for annual reports, indicative budgets and fund holding practices will be difficult to obtain for smaller groups, albeit companies, will make this available on a commercial basis. Some practices may need to amalgamate and pool their resources in order to meet the imposed requirements.

The New Contract when implemented will, undoubtedly, cause a gigantic leap forward which will raise the level of primary care. However, we must not overlook that the rationale behind the information requirements is geared to the needs for improving the hospital services and providing better value for money throughout the National Health Service.

General Practitioners are expected to continue to provide general medical services, apart from these recent commitments imposed on them. Consequently, these changes can only be achieved by a strengthening of support staff, in all disciplines, throughout general practice. If we fail to achieve this we risk making general practice an unattractive profession for future doctors.

Appendix 1

The Jarman Index

The Jarman Index, British Medical Journal, 1984.
"Under-privileged areas: Validation and Distribution of Scores".

1. Over 65s

2. Elderly living alone

3. Under 5s

4. One parent family

5. Unskilled

6. Unemployed

7. Lacking amenities

8. Overcrowding

9. Recently moved

10. Ethnic origins

Appendix 2

Information to be included in Practice Leaflets

Personal & Professional details of the Doctor(s)
Full Name
Sex
Medical qualifications
Date and place of first registration as medical practitioner

Other Information

The leaflet should indicate whether the doctor works single handed, in partnership, part time or on a job share basis, or within a group practice.

If an assistant is employed, personal details as outlined above should also be included in the practice leaflet.

If the practice is a GP training practice for the purpose of the NHS (Vocational Training) Regulations 1979(a) or undertakes the teaching of undergraduate medical students, this information needs to be included in the practice leaflet so that patients will be aware that the practice is a training practice.

cont...

Practice Information

The geographical boundary of the practice area by reference to a map of a scale approved by the FPC.

The times approved by the FPC when the doctor is available for consultation at the surgery.

Details of open and appointment systems operated by the doctor for consultation at the surgery.

Where a full appointment system is operated, the method by which a patient may obtain an URGENT or NON URGENT appointment.

The means whereby a patient obtains non urgent and urgent domiciliary visit.

Details of the system operated within the practice for patients to obtain repeat prescriptions.

Deputising arrangements for providing medical services when the doctor is not personally available.

If the practice is a dispensing practice, the arrangements for dispensing prescriptions.

Details, if appropriate, of clinics provided by the doctor including frequency, duration and purpose. This information should include information relating to whether these clinics include maternity medical services, contraceptive services, child health services and minor surgery services.

The arrangements within the practice whereby patients are able to offer comments on the provision of services.

The leaflet should also make clear that the practice premises are suitable for access by disabled patients, if not, the reasons why they are unsuitable for particular types of disability.

Appendix 3

Information to be provided in Annual Reports

1. The number of staff, other than doctors, assisting in the practice including :-

   a) the total number

   b) the main duties of each employee and the weekly hours of employment

   c) the qualifications of each employee

   d) the relevant training undertaken by each employee during the preceding 5 years

2. The following information with regard to practice premises:

   a) any variations in relation to - floor space, design, and quality, since the last Annual Report

   b) any changes planned for the forthcoming 12 month period

cont.....

3. The following information with regard to the referral of patients to other services under the NHS Act (1977) during the period of the Report :

a) Referrals by the doctor to a specialist:

      (i)   the total number of patients referred as in-patients

      (ii)   the total number of patients referred a out-patients

In each case to whichever of the following clinical specialities applies and specifying, in each case, the name of the hospital concerned.

- General Surgical

- General Medical

- Orthopaedic

- Rheumatology (Physical Medicine)

- Ear, Nose and Throat

- Gynaecology

- Obstetrics

- Paediatrics

- Opthalmology

- Psychiatry

- Geriatrics

- Dermatology

- Genito-Urinary

- Neurology

- X-Ray

- Pathology

- Others- including plastic surgery, accident & emergency and endocrinology

b) The total number of cases of which the doctor is aware(as listed above) in which a **patient referred himself / herself** to services under the NHS Act 1977

4. The doctor's other commitments as a medical practitioner :

a) a description of any post held

b) a description of work undertaken (included in this information, the annual hourly commitment)

5. The means by which the doctor or the practice staff receive patients comments on the provision of general medical services.

6. The following information with regard to order for drugs and appliances:

cont...

a) whether the doctor's practice has its own formulary

b) whether the doctor uses a separate formulary

c) the doctor's arrangements for the issues of repeat prescriptions to patients

Appendix 4

Sample letter to new entrants

Dear ....,

I would like to welcome you to .... Surgery and on behalf of the Doctors invite you to attend the Surgery for a health check. This will be undertaken by Sister .... and will include:

medical history
blood pressure check
urine examination
life-style screening

You will have every opportunity to discuss any medical problems with Sister, who will arrange for you to see Doctor if necessary.

I am enclosing a health questionnaire which I would like you to complete, as far as possible, and bring it with you to the interview.

Please come and see Sister ....
ON: ....
AT: ....
Should this be inconvenient please let me know.
Please bring a specimen of urine to this appointment.

Yours sincerely,

Practice Manager.

Appendix 5

Sample letter to patients over 75 years of age

Dear ....

I would like to extend to you an invitation to attend the
Surgery for a health check which will be undertaken by
Sister .... of the Practice Nurse Team.

Your health check will include assessment of your general
well being and you will have the opportunity to discuss any
problems you wish with Sister who will refer as necessary.

I would like you to attend Surgery :
On: Wednesday/Date ....
At: 3 p.m.
Please bring a specimen of urine.

Should the above appointment be inconvenient, please
telephone the Surgery.

Yours sincerely,

Practice Manager

Sample letter to patients due to go in of sur...

Appendix 6

Minor Surgery Procedures

Injections

Intra-articular
Peri-articular
Varicose veins
Haemorrhoids
Ganglia

Aspirations

Joints
Cysts
Bursae
Hydrocoeles
Ganglia

Incisions

Abscesses
Cysts
Perianal haematoma

Curette, cautery, cryotherapy

Warts - plantar and others
Other skin lesions

Excisions

Sebaceous cysts
Lipomata
Biopsy specimens for histology
Intra-dermal
     naevi
     papillomata
     dermatofibromata
     rodent ulcers
Warts
Ganglia
Toe nails

Others

Vasectomy
Removal of foreign bodies
Varicose veins - ligation
Nasal cautery